I0428214

JPM
Oral Hygiene protocol

Chapters 9 & 10 (TEN PAGES) taken from the

NCD
Flaxseed Shake
recipe
(Not Included)
(available online)

Jumper Publications and Media

Disclaimer

The purpose of this book is to empower the reader with knowledge, to educate, informational purposes. This book is not medical advice, but rather the author's personal experience, and is a guide for anyone who wishes to implement said dietary or lifestyle changes at the reader's own discretion. The choice between medical care and self care is completely up to the reader. If you have a medical problem, seek medical care. The author and Jumper Publications and Media shall not be held responsible or liable for any and all damages, loss, or injury, of any kind that may be caused or allegedly caused, directly or indirectly, by the information in this book. Reading beyond this page is the reader's consent to the above disclaimer.

Other Publications

ABC Water and the Number Crunch Diet
a step by step solution to alkaline deficiency and
with a New and Unique approach to weight control

Nontoxic Teeth Whitening and Dental Hygiene System
"Spare me the chemicals, I've switched to FOOD GRADE to
whiten, gargle and brush."

NCD Flaxseed Shake Recipe
the Number Crunch Diet method for getting omega 3s
and with three variations so you'll never get bored

12 Changes A Year – Volume 1
the recipe book to the Number Crunch Diet
When you take control of the numbers
you take control of your weight.

The 5 Points of Posture
the missing link to fat loss, overall wellness, and
to becoming Respected, Adored, and Wealthy

12 Changes A Year – Volume 2
the recipe book to the Number Crunch Diet
Begin today and forever be in control of the numbers you're eating.

Vision Is Possible
Improve your vision and get a facelift for free!
an original vision program targeting your Eye Lids

To purchase additional copies, please visit

http://www.CreateSpace.com/5015931

CONTENTS

Edits & Format

You will notice oddities in punctuation, spelling, syntax, and perhaps even semantics, within this book. Feel free to let me know, but some of it is done for brevity or to shift emphasis. I use capitals where I see fit, to grab your attention and make it stand out, and I also remove capitals when I don't think they are deserving of them, or to remove emphasis after first usage, i.e., Pyrex becomes pyrex. And french bread, brussels sprouts, and english cucumbers, are spelled lowercase, as we are not going to "link" a European vacation to our food and eating.

Secondly, I will unhyphenate to create rhythm. Grammatically, two or more words that function as an adjective before a noun are supposed to be hyphenated. That's fine. A million-dollar smile, is the adjective "million-dollar" describing the smile. However, this can get redundant after a while, 1&2 3, 1&2 3, 1&2 3. The noun gets all the attention. But what if you want the adjectives to have the emphasis? After all, the adjectives are the descriptive words. So, I will drop the hyphens to allow the adjectives equal emphasis, and to change the pace of the sentence a bit. So if there are no hyphens, read it slower and evenly, one two three four five six seven. A "step-by-step solution" sounds a bit skippy and simplistic, whereas, a "step by step solution" is said slower and sounds more methodical. Hyphenating two words, or joining two words as a compound word, reduces their individual meanings.

With regard to fastfood, healthfood, and seasalt, it's time for these words to evolve into compound words, so the trend starts here.

There are also some fragmented sentences, subject-verb disagreements, and singular/plural violations. When "correcting" certain of these sentences, they lost their emphasis and punch, so I kept them as is.

In the past I've been guilty of judging other author's sentences, only to reread it with the commas, pauses, and then it made perfect sense. So, if there's a comma, then pause, as you may not get to pause later in the sentence. If there's no comma, then don't pause and read it all as one.

I pose questions, but without question marks. Some are rhetorical, but some are to make you Ponder. Great word. Ponder. If you see a question mark at the end, then it requires an answer. If there's no question mark, then you can just say, yeah, no, or hm.

English continues to change, people using it, customize the language to fit what they want to communicate, emphasize, and to make their point from various angles. It also has to have a variety of melodies and rhythms to keep it from being boring. If you find yourself having to reread a sentence, it may be that it's structured that way for that very reason. So take your time. Don't rush. Let the words digest, so that you absorb the material, and hopefully take some of it and make it a part of your life.

Lastly, you will notice that I customized the headers of every page! This is not something Microsoft Word Starter allows you to do. You can only customize three pages, first, even, and odd. So, to get around this I had to create a Page Break every three pages, and as a result, the last line of some of the pages doesn't "justify" to the edge. So I hope that flipping through the upper corners of the pages will assist you in finding the chapter that you are looking for.

You won't see any citations from scientific studies or PubMed, because at JPM we look to a higher source for our reference.

God Bless!

Enjoy the Journey

Email me if you have a question, or if you just want to comment. Your purchase comes with 3-months free support and photos.

Barry Ogston, B.Sc., CLS, MLS(ASCP)

You have to crunch the numbers to see what you're really eating.

CHAPTER 9

JPM Mouth Rinse Protocol™

In the highly competitive world of publishing and creating a following, a reader base, you've always got to give your audience something for free. This way, if the book was not quite what they thought it was worth, the "free" item will hopefully make up for it. Keep in mind, I price things according to what I would pay for them and according to other things. People pay $250 to see a sporting event, but squawk about the price of information that can positively affect their health for decades to come. A one-night stay in your average hotel room while on vacation can cost $179, and it's long gone. Someone told me he sold a used fishing lure on eBay for $400. What's really going to help you on your journey?

As a lifetime seeker of self-improvement, I have never thought twice about the price if I knew it would benefit me. I left Timothy Ferris, author of *The Four Hour Body*, a 5-star review, even though I had to read all 572 pages of his book to get two things out of it. But, it's two things that I didn't have before I read the book. A person with a lot of these Gold Nuggets is miles ahead in the game of life than someone who just goes along never seeking information. So, there's your good advice. And if you are curious to know what those two things are that I got from his book, stay tuned!

Okay, I'll tell you.

This may not be new to some of you but it was to me.

1. Glut Ham Raises – totally works the backs of your legs.

Not just the hamstrings but the calves and butt as well. Attempt to do 12-15 slow reps in 60 seconds and you will feel it the next day. Best bang for your Back-Of-The-Leg buck. However, for erectors, inner hip muscles, I still like single leg "rocking" deadlifts.

2. MED – Minimal Effective Dose
It's best explained like this. Water comes to a boil when it reaches 100 degrees celsius. Adding more heat, more energy, doesn't make it boil more. Applying this to exercise, it's the old "Stimulate Don't Annihilate" rule. Do one set to failure and that's it. Stop. You're done. Let your muscles break down and regrow bigger. It works. And the best part is, you keep cortisol levels under control. Heavy workouts can zap your body for days, especially when you're over 50!

So this is why *ABC Water and the Number Crunch Diet* is priced like a BMW. It's Revelation Information. A synergy of dozens of books and specialties, to create a completely new book. Selfcare.

So your free report is about "How To Improve Your Gums And Teeth". Two words. Hydrogen Peroxide.

But not so fast. There's the detail.

JPM Mouth Rinse Protocol™

I have to give credit to my brother for this one. He is 62, has never had a cavity, and 33-years ago his dentist told him that he doesn't need to keep coming to the dentist, that, "You're your own dentist."

Now, how many people do you know of that have been told by their dentist that their personal dental hygiene is so good that they are their own dentist and that the dentist actually tells them to stop coming to the dentist? I only know of one. My brother. And he has fantastic teeth and gums, and he's 62, retirement age. What was his secret weapon all these years. Hydrogen Peroxide.

I recall a coworker telling me she had so many dental problems and she was so upset about them. I told her to rinse with hydrogen peroxide. She came back the next week with a big smile on her face, all that anxiety that she had was gone, and she sincerely thanked me profusely. She was smiling bigger and I could tell her gums were looking better already.

Lack of Attached Gingiva. Nobody wants to hear their dentist or dental hygienist say this. Gingiva just means gums. Lack of attached gums, means you have pockets. You know, like when they do the probing of your gums, 334 333 233 432. They go around your teeth checking the pockets of your gums at three locations on each tooth, cheek side and tongue side. Bleeding and pockets means GINGIVITIS. Gum Disease. Bad News.

But there's hope. You can, in my experience, and obviously in my brother's experience, have healthy gums by rinsing with hydrogen peroxide. But there's some do's and don'ts, so keep reading.

I will give you the whole protocol that I do so that you can set it up for yourself at home and begin today to drop those pocket measurements from four and three millimeters to two and one millimeters, and yes, it is possible to have zero mm pockets. Zero mm pockets means you have 100% fully-attached gums to your teeth. My brother has this. You can tell when he smiles. He's got solid gums that are gripped solidly on to his teeth. No pockets. No recession. No Lack of Attached Gingiva.

Of course we have all asked him where he got the idea to rinse with hydrogen peroxide. His answer is brilliant.

"I just thought, well, I'll rinse with hydrogen peroxide."

You see, you don't have to be a doctor to know things, or a PhD, or a licensed blah blah blah. My brother is none of those things. Yet he's a genius when it comes to oral hygiene. AND, the most notable part of his discovery is, It Just Came To Him. Like a thought. Or a revelation. He already had a million-dollar smile, so he was thinking about how he could maintain it and improve on it so that he could have that million dollar big teeth square jaw smile for his whole life.

Imagine having perfect teeth and gums and you haven't been to the dentist in 33 years. In the ABC NCD book I talk about not paying too much attention to crossover double-blind placebo-controlled scientific studies. For some things, the obvious answer is right in front of your face. Just look and believe it. I don't need a study to prove to me that hydrogen-peroxide rinsing can transform bad gum tissue into healthy gum tissue and reduce pocket depth. I use it and it does it. Every one of our family members uses it. We are all following my brother's oral hygiene protocol.

So, here's what you do.

Initial Setup. Buy 8 bottles of 15oz Lea & Perrins Worcestershire sauce at the supermarket. Transfer the liquid to a one-gallon container, or discard it, then proceed to thoroughly rinse the bottles and scrub off the labels. Now you have eight 15oz glass amber bottles with tight-fitting screw caps. The amber color will prevent light from degrading the H_2O_2 into water, and the screw cap will prevent oxygen from getting inside and reacting with the H_2O_2 and converting it into water. So your hydrogen peroxide will stay potent. Also, if you haven't already read my website, we here at JPM and ABC NCD are Plastiphobes. We avoid plastics for eating and for anything that will go in our mouth or used on our body. The HUGE one is, never microwave food in a plastic container, and the lesser evils are, storing the shampoo you use on your head in a plastic container. Replace the plastic containers in your kitchen and bathroom with glass wherever possible.

So, this 15oz bottle is ideal and you'll see why as we go along.

Next. Buy a gallon of hydrogen peroxide. I get mine at Smart & Final supermarket and restaurant-supply store, $8. It's the most economical, $1 per 16oz. And a gallon will keep you from running out. Fill your eight worcester bottles full to the top, to the brim, and then cap them. The bottle holds 16oz exactly, so you have the exact amount needed to fill all 8 bottles to the top. If the bottles were really only 15oz, then 8x15=120oz, and a gallon is 128oz, so you would have 8oz left over. BUT, lucky for you, I have already figured out the perfect bottle.

The other reason for using this bottle is because it has a small mouth. You want to be able to control the amount of hydrogen peroxide entering your mouth as you take a "swig". A wide-mouth bottle will have you pouring in too much H_2O_2 into your mouth. This is important because:

1. Hydrogen peroxide is for external use only. Don't Drink it.
2. If you get too much in your mouth, and it makes contact with the back of your throat, your throat will dry out and you'll end up with a raspy voice.

That brings us to the Technique.
Pucker your lips and use your tongue to control the liquid as it enters your mouth.   When you have about a tablespoon of hydrogen peroxide in your mouth, half an ounce, close your lips and use your cheeks to swirl the liquid around your teeth and gums.

DON'T LET IT TOUCH THE BACK OF YOUR MOUTH

You will have a raspy voice and dry throat if you do.

H_2O_2 IS NOT FOR GARGLING

I will tell you what to use for oral gargling at the end. Your Second Free Report!

So with the H_2O_2 in your mouth, swirl for 30 seconds minimum or 60 seconds maximum. Any less than 30s and you're not doing it long enough for cleaning action to occur, and any longer than 60s and it's no longer doing anything because it's all deactivated, reacted.

Until you get comfortable with this technique, keep your chin down. The natural reaction is to gargle as you are swirling. Don't.

KEEP YOUR CHIN DOWN in the beginning. After a month, the habit should be solidified and you will be able to keep your head in its natural upright position and multitask or stare at yourself in the mirror as you swirl. Are you looking HYA??

Place one of your worcester 16oz hydrogen-peroxide bottles in the shower for your morning oral-hygiene routine, and place the other in the medicine cabinet above your bathroom sink for your before-bed oral-hygiene routine.

16oz will last about one month, 1T, or half an ounce, times 30 days. So, once a month you will start a new bottle in the shower and a new bottle in the medicine cabinet. This is why eight bottles and the one gallon of hydrogen peroxide is the way to do it. When you run out, you just grab another bottle. Two bottles a month means that your eight bottles will last you four months. So every 4 months, or 16 weeks, 3 times a year, you have to pick up a gallon of H_2O_2 and aliquot it into your eight bottles. This is your system.

I gave a bottle to a friend and he freaked out because his gums were foaming up. I said, "Yeah, your gums are foaming up because your gum lines are dirty." He did it twice a day and on the third day they just foamed up a small normal amount. He thanked me profusely.

And I do mean profusely. People are amazed at how amazing this works for reversing bad gums and for making them look that healthy pink color. And no more sensitive areas after a while.

And I've NEVER heard this anywhere. I honestly believe that when this goes viral, mainstream, because of its effectiveness, that the originator was my brother, back in the 1970s, when something, God maybe, inner Divine Intelligence maybe, said, "I think I'll try rinsing with hydrogen peroxide."

You heard it here first. But the credit goes to my brother Ken!

CHAPTER 10

JPM Mouth Wash Protocol™

This next one, I will take credit for. And that's the mouth rinse for gargling, aka, mouth wash.

You know, I've never liked using mouthwash. Whenever I tried it, you know, the typical brand they advertise on TV that starts with the letter L, my eyes would get red and my mouth would burn and I'd spit it out and ask myself.

"Why does mouthwash have to feel so toxic?"

Well, fast-forward to the modern world and we now know that IT IS TOXIC. It's loaded with toxic cancer causing birth defect inducing hormone disrupting CHEMICALS!

You will never convince me that thymol, eucalyptol, methyl salicylate, menthol, alcohol, benzoic acid, poloxamer 407, and caramel, are safe and essential for oral hygiene. Salicylate is aspirin. Why does mouthwash need aspirin? To calm the inflammatory effect from all the chemicals.

And that "alcohol", well, it doesn't say if it's ethanol, the drinkable one, but it could be isopropyl alcohol, rubbing alcohol, the poisonous one, or it could be a mixture of the two. Dr. Hulda Clark in her book, *The Cure For All Diseases*, states that she detects isopropyl alcohol contamination everywhere in our lives because the food industry uses it to sanitize. So the next morning they start up the food-processing machines and all that isopropyl alcohol residue ends up in the food. In trace amounts and randomly, yes, but when you are getting exposed to it from every angle, it begins to build up in the body. She stated in her book that every single cancer patient is toxic with isopropyl alcohol.

There's a group of people who bash her books, and I am not saying she was 100% spot-on with every word she wrote, no person is, and she often said when interviewed that, "We haven't discovered that part yet." But her 604-page book is packed with information and it's the reason that today you hear about pollutants, contamination, chemicals, toxins, detox, and purity. I highlighted and underlined more than half of the book and it took me six months to read it.

So although I take credit for this mouthwash, I really need to give credit to the late Dr. Hulda Clark and *The Cure For All Diseases*. You see, vodka is food-grade alcohol. It's the only food-grade alcohol. And alcohol is a good germ-killer, sanitizer, cleaner, and antiseptic.

JPM Mouth Wash Protocol™

Buy a 1.75 liter bottle of vodka, 40% alcohol by volume, not 25%.

I used to buy the Heritage brand 1.75L 40% vodka at Albertson's supermarket for $9.99, $8.99 on sale, plus tax, but the bottle is plastic.

Plastiphobe

So now I buy the "UV" brand 40% vodka in the 1.75L glass bottle. It's $16.99 at Albertson's, but other grocery stores stock it as well.

I spent a while deciding which glass bottle of vodka to go with, and the UV brand won, as the glass is clear, the shape is smooth, and it has indentations at the back for your hand to grip it. Nice.

40% is too strong for gargling so you will want to dilute it 50/50 half-and-half with water. Go to the healthfood store and buy a few bottles of bottled water in glass. Drink the water and remove the labels. I use Voss brand 400mL cylindrical glass water bottles with screw caps.   Nice and classy looking when you get the label cleaned off. Place the bottle on your scale and turn it on. Add 200 grams of vodka, then add 200 grams of water. Voila, 20% vodka.

This is your mouthwash for gargling.

As with the worcester bottles, buy eight Voss water bottles so that you have some ready-to-use when you run out. I use this 20% alcohol to rinse my mouth after meals during the day, along with flossing and brushing. For toothpaste I use Trader Joe's/Tom's brand, with Fennel, Propolis and Myrrh, lavender color on the box.

Tom's brand has been around for a long time and back in the 1980s is was the only Health Food toothpaste. In the 1990s they used to put the PURPOSE for their ingredients on the toothpaste box. So, they had a list of about six ingredients in one column, and the purpose for each ingredient right across from it in another column. They stopped doing this. Now they just list the ingredients, and shockingly, GLUTAMATE is ingredient number seven.   This is why I don't use toothpaste that frequently. Glutamate, Excitotoxin, is in my Health Food toothpaste. Terrible.

JPM Oral Hygiene AM Protocol™
Brush – toothpaste
Floss
Mouth Rinse – 1T H_2O_2 30-60sec
Mouth Wash – 20% vodka gargle & rinse 10-15sec

Throughout the day and after eating:
Brush – no toothpaste
Floss
Mouth Wash – 20% alcohol gargle and rinse

JPM Oral Hygiene BB Protocol™
Before Bed same as AM

Hard/Firm toothbrush if my tongue feels a gritty film anywhere. Scaling tool once a week on anterior lowers (minerals in my saliva tend to precipitate on the backs of my lower teeth). And I use one of those long Oral B-60 toothbrushes to clean my tongue AM and PM. A lot of people neglect their tongue hygiene.

If you don't already own one, a Must-Have is an electric toothbrush. Hand brushing simply can't compare to the fast vibrating movement of an electric toothbrush. Philips Sonicare $35, works great. I keep one in my car. (No that's not weird.)

I am not as fortunate as my brother in that I still go to get my teeth cleaned every 6-12 months, but my hygienist and dentist always remark at how good my gums look, and how clean my teeth are. Apparently, a lot of teenagers have poor gum health and oral hygiene. Soft drinks! It's liquid sugar. The NCD considers soda pops as poisons, especially acidic colas. They're Anti-Nutrition. Health destroying.

Recall from the ABC NCD that – No amount of good can counter the bad you expose yourself to daily. You've got to eliminate the bad. In the old days, I can remember coke being used to remove the corroded-metal buildup from the posts of a car battery. And it worked good. Think about what it's doing to your teeth and gums.

As a final note, my next project is to discontinue using 3% topical hydrogen peroxide from the body-care aisle, and order 35% food-grade hydrogen peroxide from www.purehealthdiscounts.net. Then, just dilute it to about 3% by adding 1.5 ounces of the 35% H_2O_2 to the worcester bottle and then filling it to the top with water. See *Nontoxic Teeth Whitening and Dental Hygiene System*

And as another word of caution regarding the use of hydrogen peroxide as a mouth rinse.

IT'S NOT RECOMMENDED IF YOU HAVE METAL FILLINGS.

The H_2O_2 will, on a small scale, dissolve the metal, and those metal atoms can then be absorbed into your bloodstream via the capillary beds underneath your tongue, causing you to auto-intoxicate yourself over time. But if you have metal fillings in your mouth, your saliva is doing the same thing to a lesser degree 24-hours-a-day 7-days-a-week. If it was me, I would still do the hydrogen-peroxide mouth rinse AM and PM, as the benefits of having attached gingiva and healthy gums outweighs the risk of trace amounts of metal dissolving, getting into the bloodstream, and traveling to various locations within the body. Best advice is to have them removed and redone with composite, PLASTIC!

As a benefit to using the H_2O_2 mouth rinse AM and PM, you'll have nice white teeth! Peroxide is the active ingredient in most teeth whiteners.

Hope You Enjoyed This.

Jumper Publications & Media
Your First Choice for Selfcare

Once you've set up these two oral hygiene protocols and begin to see the benefits for yourself, why not hit the website and purchase a copy for a friend or family member, boss, coworker or your employees. For $30 you could purchase 10 copies and hand them out as "thank-you" tokens to people you know. Remember, it's fully copyrighted ISBN 978-1502489142 so making copies and free distribution is illegal – and bad Karma!

PREVIEW
from the
ABC Water and the Number Crunch Diet

As you know, the recipes for the NCD are being published under the titles, *12 Changes a Year* – the companion guide to the Number Crunch Diet. It may take up to a year to get them written as it will comprise about three volumes. In the meantime, you can get your pH paper testing set up and determine your current alkaline stores. The recipes read like a book and include additional information that I've discovered about diet, lifestyle, health and selfcare. I look forward to seeing you over there!

To join my mission in providing people with safe, effective, affordable, selfcare protocols, send someone you know to www.abcwaterandthenumbercrunchdiet.com. Tell them to take the Quiz!! Thanks for your support! God Bless.

Jumper Publications & Media
from Advice to Results

I almost forgot! (again, not really) to tell you!

If you liked this shake recipe be sure to check out

TCY
12 Changes a Year
Vol 2

for the NCD ORANGE SHAKE!
It makes 9, and I often repeat the recipe midweek.
And whey protein – but not from powder.

BUY THE BOOK!!
IT'S GOOD STUFF!

Leave a Review

Without giving away the secret protocols, "spoilers", recommend this publication and leave a review so that someone else might benefit from it too. Thank you.

www.amazon.com   Search: Oral Hygiene Protocol

Subscribe to my YouTube Channel
www.youtube.com   Search: Number Crunch Diet

Be sure to send me an email so I can periodically keep in touch with updates and new Selfcare Strategies – and discount offers on new items (yes, more than books!) (a simple and effective weight-loss device) (weightlifting "device" that I use EVERY time I work out) and don't forget the recipes! – TCY.

abcwaterandthenumbercrunchdiet@mail.com
Privacy – your email address will not be used for anything other than by Jumper Publications and Media.

FOLLOW-UP

You know, I've never liked the idea of brushing with baking soda because I've had in my mind all these years a picture of my dad brushing his teeth with the white-and-blue box of Arm & Hammer baking soda, and I assumed it was the one from the cleaning products aisle, which has contaminants and is too abrasive.

So, that glutamate in my toothpaste, and the fact that something in me, my Divine Intelligence, is telling me it's not good, has led me to rethink the baking soda for brushing.

Well, here's what you do. Buy baking soda in the BAKING aisle at a good-quality supermarket, I buy mine at Trader Joe's Market and it's USP, United States Pharmacopeia grade, the highest grade you can buy. To a 16oz glass jar, add the entire contents of the baking soda, use it to brush your teeth. Just wet the bristles and touch the powder, brush for two minutes, works great. Just the right amount of abrasion, not too rough not too mild. The food-grade USP baking soda in the baking aisle is so finely ground it's like a light soft powder, Perfect. The baking soda also gives your body a slight amount of bicarbonate, sodium bicarbonate, for alkalinity. See *ABC Water and the Number Crunch Diet* for the significance of alkalinity to good health, energy, and being ailment free.

So the JPM Oral Hygiene Protocol™ becomes,

1. food-grade or USP-grade baking soda to brush
2. 3% topical or food-grade hydrogen peroxide for gum lines
3. 20% food-grade vodka to gargle

The hydrogen peroxide and the baking soda will whiten.

If you do buy the 35% hydrogen peroxide, dilute it to 6% instead of 3% for a super-powerful teeth whitener! However, if you just be consistent and do the hydrogen-peroxide mouth rinse protocol AM and PM every day, you won't need more whitener. The 3% twice a day works perfectly. Happy Hygiene!

Saliva vs Urine pH

Top Ten Reasons Why Saliva pH Is Worthless When Compared To Urine pH For Acid-Base Analysis

#10 Small Volume – small tiny volume samples don't represent the whole

#9 Difficult to Obtain – the procedure is to bring up saliva and swallow, 2x, then use the third one for the test, too hard to obtain

#8 Poor Reproducibility – when you retest your saliva sample, you will likely get a slightly different color (reading)

#7 Poor Accuracy – if you collect a second sample, it will likely give you a different reading than the first

#6 Bacterial Contamination – bacteria from your mouth will interfere with the test

#5 Food Contamination – food from your mouth will interfere with the test

#4 Spoon Contamination – the surface of the spoon that you collect it on is going to affect your small sample

#3 Viscosity – saliva is too thick and results in faded or dual colors of the test pad (or paper)

#2 Difficulty Reading – the color doesn't "lock in" so you can take a reading, it tends to change shades through a range

#1 Your Salivary Glands have ZERO to do with Acid-Base regulation. Try Kidneys.

Your kidneys are running your body's alkaline status.

And your alkaline status is the secret they don't want you to know.

Pick the correct answers – There may be more than one

1. A urine pH of 5 is telling you
   a. about your blood pressure
   b. that you're tired
   c. about your alkaline reserves
   d. to see a doctor
   e. that you're healthy and fine

2. Urine pH testing is routinely performed by licensed
   a. social workers
   b. clinical laboratory scientists
   c. respiratory therapists
   d. fitness advisors
   e. nurses and doctors

3. The cost of one month of urine pH testing is _____ the cost of open heart surgery (CABG).
   a. 1/10
   b. 1/100
   c. 1/1000
   d. 1/10,000
   e. 1/100,000

4. The opposite of metabolic acid is dietary
   a. phosphates – found in meats and cola drinks
   b. bicarbonate – found in packaged foods
   c. caffeine – found in green tea
   d. bicarbonate – found in fruits and vegetables
   e. bicarbonate – found in oils and fats

5. Information can be of which types
   a. true
   b. incomplete

c. false
d. clouded
e. secret

6. "Natural Flavor" on a food label is
   a. natural flavor extracts from plants and fruit
   b. glutamates, MSG, altered salts
   c. chemicals that make you addicted to the product
   d. generally safe and good for me
   e. not something I need to worry about

7. During World War II, the people who failed to act early
   a. suffered
   b. died
   c. lost everything
   d. became victims
   e. made it through unscathed

8. Compensating means
   a. saving for retirement
   b. eating foods that lift your mood
   c. doing something to mask something
   d. brushing it out of your thoughts
   e. pleasing others and being a do-gooder
   f. all of the above

9. The reason(s) people are fat
   a. they're born that way
   b. they don't make their own meals
   c. hereditary – handed down from your parents
   d. my body just won't lose fat
   e. they don't see the numbers in what they're eating

10. The "Cheat Day" is
    a. a great way to get food cravings satisfied
    b. required to reset my fat-burning hormones
    c. a 2-8 step backwards day
    d. works well for most people long term
    e. is a popular "trick" that you should buy into

ANSWERS

1. A urine pH of 5 is telling you
    a. about your blood pressure – No, but there is a relationship
       (see Chapter 24)
    b. that you're tired – No, but there is a relationship (see Chapter
       20)
    c. about your alkaline reserves – YES! Get to know your
       alkaline status by reading this book.
    d. to see a doctor – No, but it can lead to that.
    e. that you're healthy and fine – One number tells you little, 35
       numbers a week tells you a lot. Get to know your urine pH.

2. Urine pH testing is routinely performed by licensed
    a. social workers – no
    b. clinical laboratory scientists – Yes, 99% of all urine testing is
       done by a CLS.
    c. respiratory therapists – no
    d. fitness advisors – no
    e. nurses and doctors – Doctors do perform urine tests in their
       offices, but they are not looking at urine pH with much depth.

3. The cost of one month of urine pH testing is _____ the cost of
   open heart surgery (CABG)(a bypass, "cabbage").
    a. 1/10 – no
    b. 1/100 – no
    c. 1/1000 – no
    d. 1/10,000 – Yes. You can test all of your urinations for about

$1 a month (see Chapter 11). A cabbage would run you at least $10,000.
   e. 1/100,000 – no. But I believe the potential to save yourself $100,000 in medical treatments is very possible.

4. The opposite of metabolic acid is dietary
   a. phosphates – no, phosphates contribute to acidity
   b. bicarbonate – no, bicarbonate yes, but not from packaged foods
   c. caffeine – no, caffeine is a drug, most drugs are acidic
   d. bicarbonate found in fruits and vegetables – Yes!
   e. bicarbonate found in oils and fats – no, oils and fats are not sources of bicarbonate

5. Information can be of which types
   a. true – Yes, this is a bit what your life is all about. Finding the truth about things.
   b. incomplete – aka, partial truths or half truths, aka, "spin". Do you find your head spinning when you go for fancy medical treatments?
   c. false – lies, yes lies. Don't call them untruths. Lies are Lies. When people lie it's your job to call them on it. Otherwise, "ya got no backbone".
   d. clouded – blurry, muddied, confusion. I could write "scientifically" but I would just make you confused and half lost. How does that help you.
   e. secret – Now we're talking. When they say "buy this stock" you've got to be a moron to buy it. The payoffs and the winners are kept secret, shared through word of mouth.

6. "Natural Flavor" on a food label is
   a. natural flavor extracts from plants and fruit – Well, they would like you to think that, but that's far from reality.
   b. glutamates, MSG, altered salts – Yes, often this is the case.
   c. chemicals that make you addicted to the product – Yes

Absolutely
   d. generally safe and good for me – don't buy that line
   e. not something I need to worry about – you make your own
      choices in life

7. During World War II, the people that failed to act early
Referring to this is grim and bleak. But there are people suffering
and dying every day because they failed to act early. You could say
that WWII is still happening all around us in the United States of
America today. My book can help you not to fall victim to this
death and suffering. So that you make it through your life,
unscathed.

8. Compensating means
   a. saving for retirement – no, but I have seen people who are
      just a little too attached to their portfolios, compensating?
   b. eating foods that lift your mood – no, but food is commonly
      used to compensate
   c. doing something to mask something – Ah-Ha, Yes.
   d. brushing it out of your thoughts – no. It's okay and healthy to
      let go of thoughts, just be sure you're not avoiding your
      issues.
   e. people pleasing – reward seekers may be compensating
   f. all of the above – no, just C. Go back and read C again.

9. The reason(s) people are fat
   a. they're born that way – don't give me that
   b. they don't make their own meals – Bingo! This is key.
   c. heredity – your fat jeans are because of your fat genes – no I
      don't think so
   d. my body just won't lose fat – I hear you. There is not a lot of
      good help out there. Luckily, you've found the right place.
   e. they don't see the numbers in what they're eating – Yes. And
      person D above just needs to look at food mathematically
      (and read the book).

10. The "Cheat Day" is
   a. a great way to get food cravings satisfied – Wrong. I'm a testimony of getting rid of food cravings. See Chapter 38, 39, 40, 41.
   b. required to reset my fat-burning hormones – Wrong. If you get your macros right, your hormones will cooperate just fine.
   c. a 2-8 step backwards day – On page 84 of *The Four Hour Body* the person states that he gains 4.4 lbs on his cheat day. Then he loses it. Can you say "moody"?
   d. works well for most people long term – After reading dozens of diet books, I could not find one that worked long term, so I made my own. It's called the Number Crunch Diet.
   e. a popular "trick" that you should buy into – The Number Crunch Diet isn't about cheating. Although it's full of useful "tricks" that I came up with and use daily.

You'll be miles ahead of the average person after a while.

www.ingramcontent.com/pod-product-compliance
Lightning Source LLC
Chambersburg PA
CBHW070527290526
45790CB00003B/1338